The World of Diabetes

Reduce Your Risk for Type 2 Diabetes

Yaman Katlabi RD,

Scott Walker

2015

Table of Contents

Introduction

The spread of knowledge and technology has been a force both for good and ill, especially when it comes to our health. Although it reduced hunger, infectious disease, and poverty for millions of people, but the same social and economic shifts that have increased people's wealth have also increased the risk of developing more diseases like obesity, high blood pressure, cardiovascular disease, and diabetes.

Diabetes is a common life-long health condition. It is not an easy disease to have, it doesn't stop. Diabetes once diagnosed is for life, It is a 24/7, 365 days a year health problem.

According to National Diabetes Statistics Report, there are 29.1 million Americans, or 9.3% of the population had diabetes, 1 in 4 doesn't know.

Overall Numbers, Diabetes and Prediabetes

Data from the National Diabetes Statistics Report, 2014 (released June 10, 2014):

Prevalence: In 2012, 29.1 million Americans, or 9.3% of the population, had diabetes. Approximately 1.25 million American children and adults have type 1 diabetes.

Undiagnosed: Of the 29.1 million, 21.0 million were diagnosed, and 8.1 million were undiagnosed.

Prevalence in Seniors: The percentage of Americans age 65 and older remains high, at 25.9%, or 11.8 million seniors (diagnosed and undiagnosed).

New Cases: The incidence of diabetes in 2012 was 1.7 million new diagnoses/year; in 2010 it was 1.9 million.

Prediabetes: In 2012, 86 million Americans age 20 and older had prediabetes; this is up from 79 million in 2010.

Deaths: Diabetes remains the 7th leading cause of death in the United States in 2010, with 69,071 death certificates listing it as the underlying cause of death, and a total of 234,051 death certificates listing diabetes as an underlying or contributing cause of death.

Diabetes in Youth

- About 208,000 Americans under age 20 are estimated to have diagnosed diabetes, approximately 0.25% of that population.
- In 2008—2009, the annual incidence of diagnosed diabetes in youth was estimated at 18,436 with type 1 diabetes, 5,089 with type 2 diabetes.

What is Diabetes?

Diabetes mellitus, or diabetes, is a condition in which there is an abnormally high level of glucose in the blood because the body cannot use it properly. This is because your pancreas doesn't produce any insulin, or not enough, to help glucose enter your body's cells – or the insulin that is produced does not work properly (known as insulin resistance) because of the presence of factors that oppose the action of insulin. Many other metabolic abnormalities occur, notably an increase in ketone bodies in the blood when there is a severe lack of insulin.

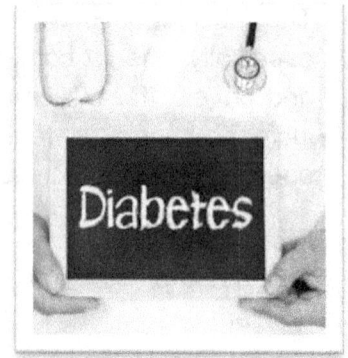

The term diabetes is the shortened version of the full name diabetes mellitus. Diabetes mellitus is derived from:

- The Greek word diabetes meaning siphon - to pass through.
- The Latin word mellitus meaning honeyed or sweet.

This is because in diabetes excess sugar is found in blood as well as the urine. It was known in the 17th century as the "pissing evil".

How Does Your Body Work?

To understand Diabetes you need to know a little more about Glucose, Insulin and Glucagon.

Glucose is a sugar and is one of the energy sources of the body. Some organs in our bodies, such as the brain, are particularly dependent upon glucose as an energy source, so it is very important that the body maintain the amount of glucose in the blood in the normal range: if the level is too high or too low, there are serious consequences. To avoid these consequences, the body has a complex set of mechanisms to keep the glucose in the normal range.

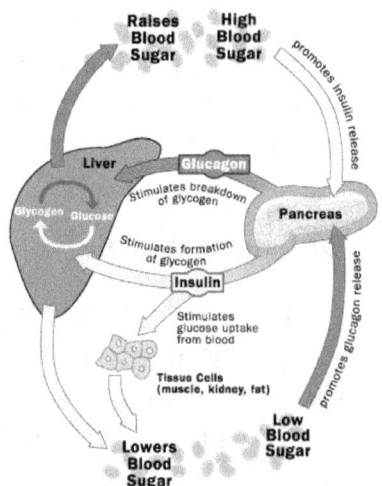

The liver is in charge of taking up and releasing glucose into the bloodstream. After a meal, the blood carrying nutrients from digestion first flows through the liver, which removes the excess glucose. When the glucose level in the blood drops (for example, after fasting or exercising), the liver does the opposite and releases glucose into the bloodstream. The liver knows how to regulate the level of glucose in the blood because it receives signals from hormones, which are chemical messengers in the blood. The two hormones that are particularly important in diabetes are insulin and glucagon.

These hormones are produced in the islets of Langerhans of the pancreas. In a person with diabetes, the beta cells which make insulin in the islets fail, and this alters the balance of insulin and glucagon actions on the tissues. The cause and degree of beta cell failure varies in different kinds of diabetes.

Insulin is the hormone that ensures that the glucose entering the bloodstream from the digestion of food is removed from the blood. Insulin also signals the body to make glycogen (a storage form of glucose) and to use glucose to make triglycerides (another important energy source) for storage in fat cells. Insulin does all this by its effects on liver cells, muscle cells, and fat cells, while Glucagon acts in an opposite manner to insulin and that balance of insulin and glucagon regulates the glucose levels in the blood during the fed and fasting states.

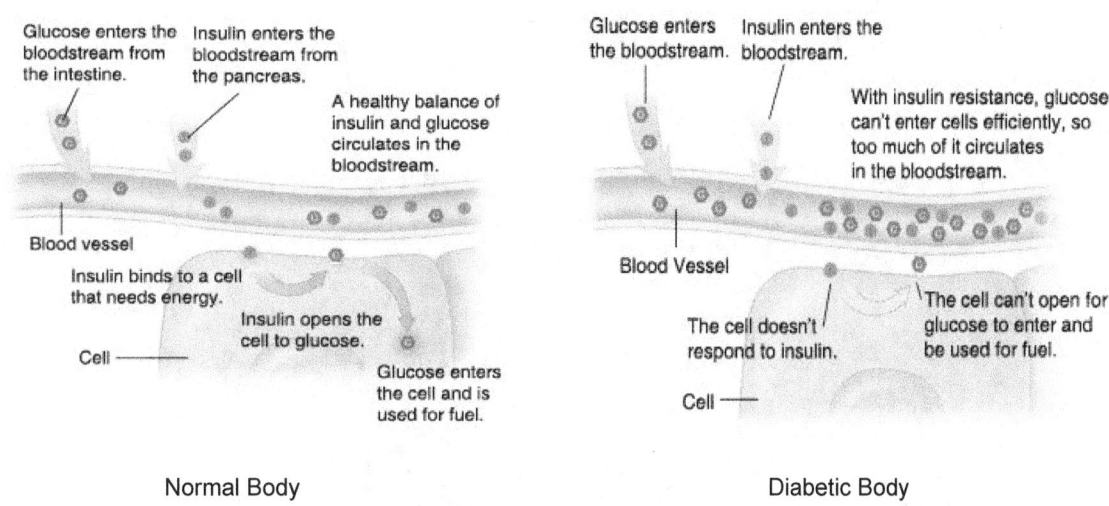

Normal Body   Diabetic Body

Signs and Symptoms of Diabetes

Depending on how high your glucose level is and how long it has been high, you may feel fairly well, or you may be so sick that you require hospitalization.

Most early symptoms are from higher-than-normal levels of glucose. One of the problems with diabetes is that the person with this disease usually feels fine and there are no symptoms. The warning signs can be so mild that he don't notice them. That's especially true of type 2 diabetes making this type of diabetes hard to detect. Some people don't find out they have it until they get problems from long-term damage caused by the disease. With type 1 diabetes, the symptoms usually happen quickly, in a matter of days or a few weeks. They're much more severe, too.

Individuals can experience different signs and symptoms, some of the signs commonly experienced include:

- Frequent urination
- Excessive thirst
- Increased hunger-even though you are eating
- Weight loss (type 1)
- loss of muscle bulk
- Extreme fatigue
- Lack of interest and concentration
- Tingling, pain, or numbness in the hands/feet (type)
- Blurred vision
- Frequent infections
- Slow-healing wounds
- Vomiting and stomach pain (often mistaken as the flu)
- Vaginal yeast infection

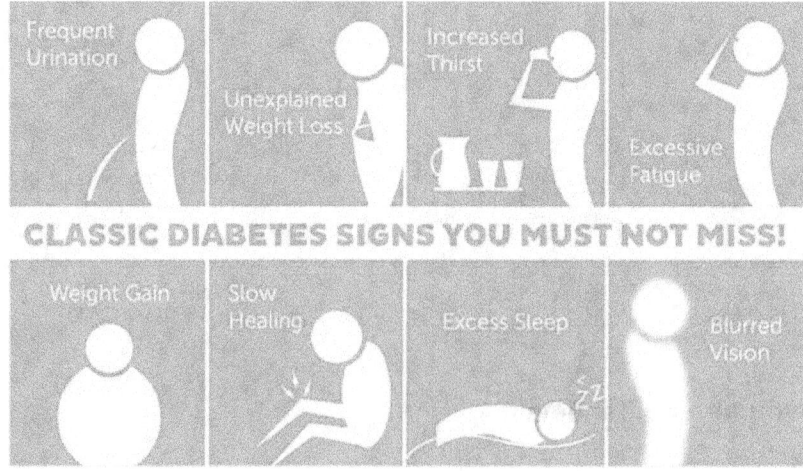

Our bodies convert the food we eat into glucose that our cells use for energy. But these cells need insulin to bring the glucose in. If our body doesn't make enough or any insulin, or if the cells resist the insulin the body makes, the glucose can't get into them and we have no energy. This can make us more hungry and tired than usual.

Normally your body reabsorbs glucose as it passes through kidneys. When you have diabetes, excess sugar (glucose) builds up in your blood. Your kidneys are forced to work overtime to filter and absorb this excess sugar. But your body may not be able to bring it all back in because your kidneys can't keep up, the excess sugar is excreted into your urine along with fluids drawn from your tissues. It will try to get rid of the extra by making more urine, and that takes fluids. This triggers more frequent urination, which may leave you dehydrated. As you drink more fluids to quench your thirst, you'll urinate even more. That is why you will pee more often and feel thirsty and tired.

Diagnosis & Normal Blood Glucose Levels

Usually, your doctor may test you for diabetes if you have previous symptoms. There are several ways to diagnose diabetes. Each way usually needs to be repeated on a second day to diagnose diabetes.

Your doctor will ask you to measure your blood glucose level. Testing should be carried out in a health care setting (such as lab). If your doctor determines that your blood glucose level is very high, or if you have classic symptoms of high blood glucose in addition to one positive test, your doctor may not require a second test to diagnose diabetes.

The following tests are used for the diagnosis of diabetes according to ADA (American Diabetes Association):

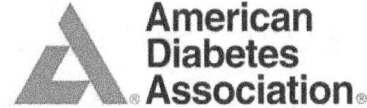

A1C

The A1C test measures your average blood glucose for the past 2 to 3 months. The advantages of being diagnosed this way are that you don't have to fast or drink anything. Diabetes is diagnosed at an A1C of greater than or equal to 6.5%.

Result	A1C
Normal	less than 5.7%
Prediabetes	5.7% to 6.4%
Diabetes	6.5% or higher

Fasting Plasma Glucose (FPG)

This test checks your fasting blood glucose levels. Fasting means not having anything to eat or drink for at least 8 hours before the test. This test is usually done first thing in the morning, before breakfast. Diabetes is diagnosed at fasting blood glucose of greater than or equal to 126 mg/dl.

Result	(FPG)
Normal	less than 100 mg/dl
Prediabetes	100 mg/dl to 125 mg/d
Diabetes	126 mg/dl or higher

Oral Glucose Tolerance Test (also called the OGTT)

The OGTT is a two-hour test that checks your blood glucose levels before and 2 hours after you drink a special sweet drink (75 grams of glucose after an overnight fast). It tells the doctor how your body processes glucose. Diabetes is diagnosed at 2 hour blood glucose of greater than or equal to 200 mg/dl.

Result	(OGTT)
Normal	less than 140 mg/dl
Prediabetes	140 mg/dl to 199 mg/dl
Diabetes	200 mg/dl or higher

Random (also called Casual) Plasma Glucose Test

This test is a blood check at any time of the day when you have severe diabetes symptoms. Diabetes is diagnosed at blood glucose of greater than or equal to 200 mg/dl.

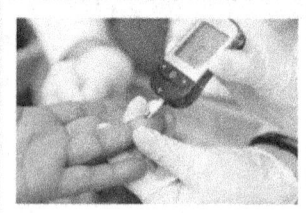

Are you at Risk?

The American Diabetes Association (ADA) has specific guidelines about who should get screened for diabetes, at what age screening should start, and what tests should be used.

- Start screening at the age of forty-five. If the test is normal, repeat every 3 years.
- Screen adults younger than forty-five if they are overweight and have one or more of the following risk factors:
    - Have a parent, sibling, or child with diabetes
    - Are physically inactive
    - Belong to an ethnic group in which there is higher risk for diabetes (African-American, Latino, Native American, Asian-American, and Pacific Islander)
    - Had diabetes during pregnancy or delivered a baby weighing more than nine pounds
    - Blood pressure readings are 140/90 or higher
    - Have an abnormal lipid profile* with a low level of HDL cholesterol (less than 35 mg/dl) and/or a high level of triglycerides (more than 250 mg/dl)

- Have a medical condition called polycystic ovary syndrome (PCOS)
- Have had previous blood glucose testing that indicated the presence of Prediabetes (described later in this chapter)
- Have circulatory problems

*A lipid panel or profile is a blood test for levels of cholesterol, triglycerides, HDL cholesterol, and LDL cholesterol.

Types of Diabetes

There are actually many different kinds of diabetes. All types of diabetes involve inadequate beta cell function, but some also involve problems with the body responding less effectively to insulin (this is known as insulin resistance). The ADA has categorized the different kinds of diabetes into four main groups:

- Type 1 diabetes
- Type 2 diabetes
- Other specific types of diabetes
- Gestational diabetes

Type 1 Diabetes

Type 1 diabetes is called insulin-dependent diabetes mellitus (IDDM) and occurs at a younger age or childhood. In these patients there is complete lack of the hormone insulin because the immune system that normally protects the body against infections goes wrong and attacks the beta cells that make insulin.

There are genetic factors and environmental factors that cause the immune system to do this. A person with this kind of diabetes has to be treated with insulin injections. Most people with this kind of diabetes are thin.

Type 2 Diabetes

Type 2 diabetes is called non-insulin dependent diabetes mellitus (NIDDM). On Type 2 the pancreas can still make insulin, but the body doesn't respond to it properly. Most people with type 2 diabetes are insulin resistant, which means they need more insulin to lower their blood glucose levels. They also have some beta cell loss in their pancreas, but not to the same extent as in type 1 diabetes. Most of the people with this kind of diabetes are overweight or obese. Genetic and environmental factors combine to cause both the insulin resistance and the beta cell loss.

It is the most common type of diabetes, around 75% of people with diabetes have type 2 diabetes mellitus. In the past, it occurred mostly in middle-aged and older individuals, but nowadays it is often seen in younger people, including children and teenagers. This number is rapidly increasing because of many factors which predisposes to type 2 diabetes.

There are more new cases of type 2 diabetes in the United States than ever before, and there are many reasons for this like overweight, obesity, high blood pressure, heart disease, low level of HDL(good cholesterol), high level of triglyceride which increases the risk for diabetes, also diabetes occurs more frequently in older individuals, and the population is aging. Ethnic minorities, especially African-Americans, Hispanics, and Asian- Americans, have a higher risk of type 2 diabetes, and there has been an increase in these populations in the United States.

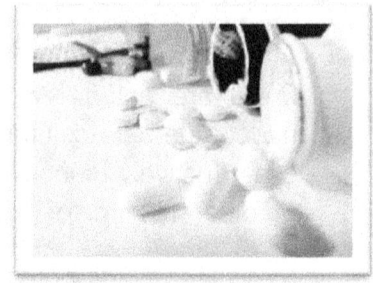

Other specific types of Diabetes

There are less common forms of diabetes in which there is a specific cause for the beta cell failure or problems with insulin function. The most common is Diabetes Due to Gene Mutations, Diabetes Due to Pancreatic Damage, Diabetes Related to Excessive Hormone Production, and Diabetes Induced by Medications.

Gestational Diabetes

Gestational diabetes occurs in pregnant women who have never had diabetes before but who have high blood sugar levels during pregnancy. Being pregnant increases the body's insulin needs. Diabetes develops when a pregnant has limited beta cell capacity and cannot respond to the additional insulin demand. Gestational diabetes affects about 4% of all pregnant women. After childbirth the mother may go on to develop type 2 diabetes.

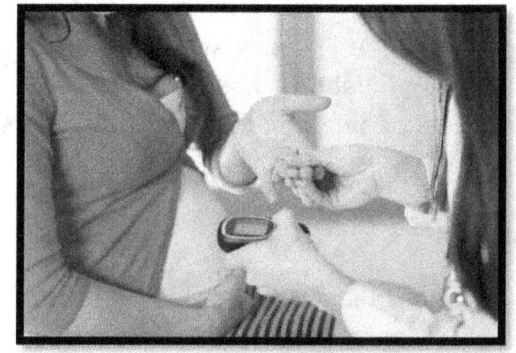

What is Prediabetes?

Before people develop type 2 diabetes, they almost always have "Prediabetes" — blood glucose levels that are higher than normal but not yet high enough to be diagnosed as diabetes.

Some people with prediabetes may have some of the symptoms of diabetes or even problems from diabetes already, while sometimes there are no clear symptoms of prediabetes, so, you may have it and not know it. According to ADA If you have prediabetes, you should be checked for type 2 diabetes every one to two years.

Complications

People with diabetes are at increased risk of serious health complications. Due to lack or insufficiency of insulin there is high blood glucose in diabetes. Excess glucose in the blood can damage the blood vessels. This leads to several complications including eye damage, vision loss, heart disease, stroke, nerve damage, DKA, hypertension, kidney failure, impotence, amputation of toes, feet or legs, and premature death.

Diabetes, when not controlled, may raise the propensity for infections. Infections and gangrene of the lower limbs is common in uncontrolled diabetes. This may necessitate an amputation if severe.

The good news, with the early detection, correct treatment and recommended lifestyle changes, many people with diabetes are able to prevent or delay the developing the complications.

Blood sugar should be regularly monitored so that any problems can be detected and treated early and will keep diabetes under control.

Diabetes Related Conditions

Hypoglycemia (Low Blood Glucose)

Hypoglycemia may also be referred to as an insulin reaction, or insulin shock. It is an important problem in type 1 diabetes, especially in patients receiving intensive therapy. It may also affect patients with type 2 diabetes who take a sulfonylurea or a meglitinide or who use insulin.

According to ADA, Hypoglycemia is a condition characterized by abnormally low blood glucose (blood sugar) levels, usually less than 70 mg/dl. However, it is important to talk to your health care provider about your individual blood glucose targets, and what level is too low for you.

Causes:

- Exercising more than normal
- Eating small portion of food
- Missing or having late meals
- Taking too much insulin or too many tablets

Signs and Symptoms (happen quickly):

- Shakiness
- Rapid/fast heartbeat
- Hunger and nausea
- Tingling lips, tongue or fingers
- Weakness or fatigue Sweating

- Headache
- Blurred /impaired vision
- Unable to speak properly

Condition Adjustment:

1. Consume 15-20 grams of glucose or simple carbohydrates.
2. Recheck your blood glucose after 15 minutes
3. If hypoglycemia continues, repeat.
4. Once blood glucose returns to normal, eat a small snack if your next planned meal or snack is more than an hour or two away.

15 grams of simple carbohydrates commonly used:

- 2 tablespoons of raisins
- 4 ounces (1/2 cup) of juice
- 1 tablespoon sugar, honey, jam or corn syrup
- 8 ounces of nonfat or 1% milk

Hyperglycemia (High Blood Glucose)

Hyperglycemia is the technical term for high blood glucose (blood sugar). High blood glucose happens when the body has too little insulin or when the body can't use insulin properly. According to ADA, If you have type 1, you may not have given yourself enough insulin or if you have type 2, your body may have enough insulin, but it is not as effective as it should be.

It can be a serious problem if you don't treat it, so it's important to treat as soon as you detect it. If you fail to treat hyperglycemia, a condition called ketoacidosis.

Ketoacidosis symptoms include: Shortness of breath, breath that smells fruity, nausea and vomiting and very dry mouth.

Causes:

- Skipping or forgetting your insulin treatments or medication
- Eating too much
- An infection anywhere in your body or illness
- Decreased activity

Signs and Symptoms:

- High blood glucose
- High levels of sugar in the urine
- Frequent urination
- Increased thirst
- Fatigue

Condition Adjustment:

- You can often lower your blood glucose level by exercising. However, if your blood glucose is above 240 mg/dl, check your urine for ketones. If you have ketones, do not exercise.
- Cut down on the amount of food and work with your dietitian to make changes in your meal plan.
- If exercise and changes in your diet don't work, your doctor may change the amount of your medication or insulin or possibly the timing of when you take it.

Prevention, treatment and care

Unfortunately, type 1 diabetes can't be prevented. Doctors can't even tell who will get it and who won't. No one knows for sure what causes type 1 diabetes, but scientists think it has something to do with genes. Eating too much sugar doesn't cause type 1 diabetes, but if you have it you should control it by taking medication that it will be insulin in the proper time, and you must keep your food choices healthy. In all type 1 diabetics and in severe uncontrolled type 2 diabetics one or more injections of insulin a day may be needed.

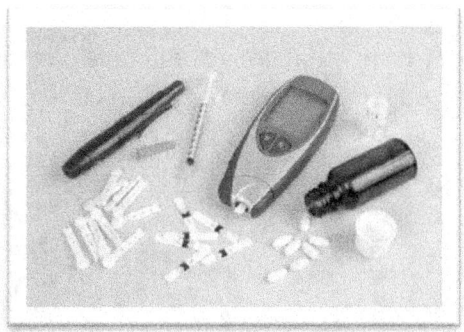

Treatment in type 2 involves both healthy diet and appropriate exercise levels as well as oral medications to regulate blood sugar.

Diabetes isn't contagious, so you can't catch it from another person.

A lot of times, taking a few safety precautions can save you some pain. So if you are a person with prediabetes or at the risk for type 2 diabetes, you can take action through everyday lifestyle habits, like exercise and healthy eating, to lower your odds of following in type 2 diabetics footsteps.

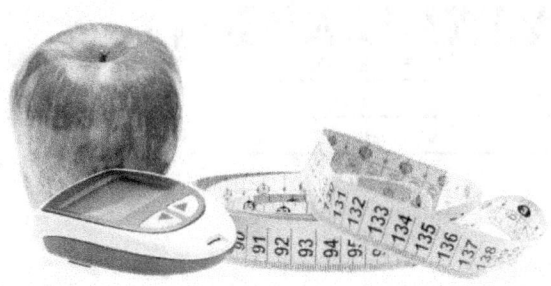

When we are talking about controlling diabetes, the following criteria must be considered:

- ✓ Ensure that symptoms have been eliminated
- ✓ Lean patients should gain weight
- ✓ Obese patients should lose weight
- ✓ Children should grow normally
- ✓ Prevention of long-term diabetic complications

Testing and recording your blood sugar levels help you see patterns you can discuss with your health care provider and other members of your diabetes care team.

Body Mass Index and Waist Circumference

BMI is a measure to estimate the degree of obesity. High BMIs are associated with increased health risks such as diabetes (Type 2) and heart diseases.

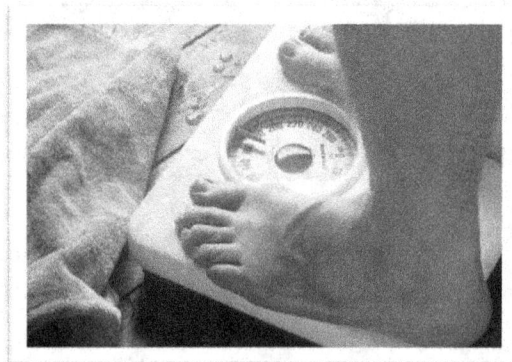

To calculate your BMI, you will need your weight and height measurements.

Formula:

Weight (kg) / [height (m)]2

The standard weight status categories associated with BMI ranges for adults are shown in the following table.

BMI	Weight Status
Below 18.5	Underweight
18.5 – 24.9	Normal
25.0 – 29.9	Overweight
30.0 and Above	Obese

But BMI is not enough to measure obesity, and it is not indicator of body fatness. The correlation between the BMI number and body fatness varies by sex, race, and age. For examples:

- ❖ At the same BMI, women tend to have more body fat than men.
- ❖ At the same BMI, older people, on average, tend to have more body fat than younger adults.
- ❖ Highly trained athletes may have a high BMI because of increased muscularity rather than increased body fatness.

BMI is only one factor related to risk for disease, we can use the circumference of the waist which is sometimes used as a simple measure of body fatness.

Adult waist circumference cut points are:

- ❖ Increased risk of health problems: Men≥ 94cm Women ≥ 80cm
- ❖ Greatly increased risk of health problems: Men ≥ 102cm Women ≥ 88cm

Let's Plan Your Meal

Healthy eating is the cornerstone of diabetic treatment and sometimes it prevents type 2 and helps to reverse prediabetes. Controlling of the diet should always be the first treatment offered to Type 2 diabetic patients before drugs are considered.

Diabetes diets typically call for portion control, carbohydrate limits and, for those who are overweight, calorie restrictions.

New understanding of the nutritional causes of type 2 diabetes gives us the power to keep it from occurring or to turn it around. Diet is not mean going hungry, healthy eating doesn't have to be difficult. Low-fat, plant-based diets are ideal for diabetes.

You can control your blood Sugar by maintain an optimal weight and pay attention to what and how much you eat.

Your dietitian can determine your ideal weight and help you to figure out how many calories you need daily and put a suitable meal plan according to your diabetes type and medications that you take.

Your body needs energy to work properly, do activities, as well as to carry out the body functions by doing the important processes of life such as breathing or growing. The amount of this energy is determined by our metabolic rate, measured in calories per day.

A calorie is a unit of energy needed to raise the temperature of 1 gram of water through 1 °C. Food that we take daily gives us these calories, the amount of these calories depends on your age, gender, size, metabolism, daily activity level and if you want to lose, maintain or gain weight.

When a person eats more calories that he need, the extra calories will be stored as a fat, so it can lead to increased weight. But if he eats fewer calories than he need his body will burn the extra fat and he will lose weight.

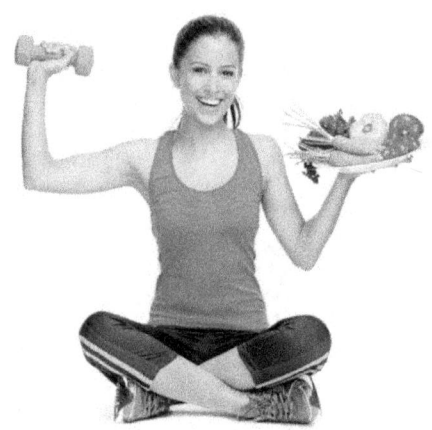

Basic Nutrients

Six basic nutrients required for good health:

1. Carbohydrates
2. Protein
3. Fat
4. Vitamins
5. Minerals
6. Water

Carbohydrates

Carbohydrates can be grouped into two categories: simple and complex. Simple carbohydrates are sugars whereas complex carbohydrates consist of starch and dietary fiber.

Carbohydrate provides about 4 kcal (kcal = kilocalories = Calories) per gram (except for fiber) and is the energy that is used first to fuel muscles and the brain. Your body can use glucose immediately or store it in your liver and muscles for when it is needed.

Simple carbohydrates include sugars found naturally in foods such as fruits, vegetables, and milk products. Simple carbohydrates also include sugars added during food processing and refining. Refined sugars are found in: biscuits, candies, raw sugar, cakes, pastries, chocolate, honey and jams, Jellies, brown and white cane sugar, pizzas, soft drinks, syrups and sweets.

Starch and dietary fiber are the two types of complex carbohydrates. Before your body can use starch as a glucose source, it must be broken down through digestion.

According to CDC, quite a few foods contain starch and dietary fiber such as breads, cereals, and vegetables:

- Starch is in certain vegetables (i.e., potatoes, dry beans, peas, and corn).
- Starch is also found in breads, cereals, and grains.
- Dietary fiber is in vegetables, fruits, and whole grain foods.

There are 2 types of fiber: Soluble and insoluble fiber. Soluble fiber lowers blood cholesterol and helps to control blood sugar levels while providing very little energy. We can find it in oat, nuts, seeds, most fruits, dry beans and peas. While we find Insoluble fiber in whole wheat bread, barley, brown rice, couscous, bulgur or whole grain cereals, wheat bran ,seeds, most vegetables, and fruits. Insoluble fiber doesn't provide any calories. It helps to alleviate digestive disorders like constipation or diverticulitis and may help prevent colon cancer. Women need 25 grams of fiber per day, and men need 38 grams per day, according to the Institute of Medicine.

Most calories (55-60%) should come from carbohydrates. Simple carbs tend to increase blood sugar mush faster than complex carbohydrates which are better for your health especially if you have diabetes or prediabetes because they take longer for your body to digest. They give you steady energy and fiber which helps you feel full.

Protein

Protein from food is broken down into amino acids by the digestive system. These amino acids are then used for building and repairing muscles, red blood cells, hair and other tissues, and for making hormones, and keeping a healthy immune system. Because protein is a source of calories (4 kcal per gram), it will be used for energy if not enough carbohydrate is available due to skipped meals, heavy exercise, etc. No more than 10-20% of calories should come from protein.

According to journal of diabetes, people with type 1 or type 2 diabetes who are in poor metabolic control may have increased protein requirements. However, the usual amount of protein consumed by people with diabetes adequately compensates for the increased protein catabolism.

Main sources of protein are animal products like meat, fish, poultry, milk, soy products, cheese and eggs and vegetable sources like legumes (beans, lentils, dried peas, nuts) and seeds

Fat

The fat in food includes a mixture of saturated and unsaturated fat. Animal-based foods such as meats and milk products are higher in saturated fat (unhealthy fat) whereas most vegetable oils are higher in unsaturated fat (the healthy fat). Nuts and some kind of fruits also contain fat like coconut and avocado.

Compared to carbohydrate and protein, each gram of fat provides more than twice the amount of calories (9 kcal per gram) but it is an essential part of our diet and nutrition, we cannot live without it. Moreover, there is some vitamins which soluble in fat and don't soluble in water. Fat maintains skin and hair, cushions vital organs, provides insulation, and is necessary for the production and absorption of certain vitamins and hormones.

ADA recommends of trying to eat less saturated and trans fat — the unhealthy fats to lower the risk of heart disease, At the same time, you can protect your heart by eating more mono and polyunsaturated fats including omega-3s — the healthy fats which lower the LDL (bad cholesterol) and raise the HDL (the good cholesterol).

Omega-3 fatty acids are found in fish, soybean products, walnuts, and flaxseeds.

Sources of monounsaturated (good or healthy) fats include: avocado, canola oil, nuts like (almonds, cashews, pecans, and peanuts), olive oil and olives, peanut butter and peanut oil sesame seeds.

Foods containing saturated fat (unhealthy fat) include high-fat meats like regular ground beef, bologna, hot dogs, sausage, bacon and spareribs, high-fat dairy products such as full-fat cheese, cream, ice cream, whole milk, butter, coconut and coconut oil, palm oil, poultry skin (chicken and turkey).

Sources of cholesterol include: high-fat dairy products (whole or 2% milk, cream, ice cream, full-fat cheese), egg yolks, liver and other organ meats, high-fat meat and poultry skin.

Food product labels will often list the total amount of fat they contain, including saturated, monounsaturated, polyunsaturated, and trans fats. Although not all fat is a source of cholesterol, all fat is high in calories. For people with and without diabetes no more than 35 percent of daily calories should come from fat and no more than 10% of energy as saturated fat.

Vitamins

Vitamins are essential micronutrients your body needs in small amounts for various roles throughout the human body. There are 13 Vitamins divided into two groups: water-soluble (B-complex vitamins and C vitamins) and fat-soluble vitamins (A, D, E and K). Without enough vitamins and minerals, your body could contract serious diseases.

The body can't make vitamins, so we have to obtain them through the diet. Many people say that they feel more energetic after consuming vitamins, but vitamins are not a source of energy (calories). Vitamins are best consumed through a varied diet rather than as a supplement because there is little chance of taking too high a dose.

Minerals

Minerals are components of foods that are involved in many body functions. There are two kinds of minerals: macro minerals and trace minerals. Macro minerals are minerals your body needs in larger amounts. They include calcium, phosphorus, magnesium, sodium, potassium, and chloride. Your body needs just small amounts of trace minerals. These include iron, copper, iodine, zinc, fluoride, and selenium.

For example, calcium and magnesium are important for bone structure, and iron is needed for our red blood cells to transport oxygen. Like vitamins, your body can't make minerals and they are not a source of energy and are best obtained through a varied diet rather than supplements.

Water

Water is a vital nutrient for good health. Most of our body weight (60-70%) is made up of water. Water helps to control our body temperature, helps energize muscles and maintain the balance of body fluids, keep skin looking good, maintain normal bowel function, carries nutrients and waste products from our cells, and is needed for our cells to function. It is recommended that adults drink 8-10 glasses of fluid daily (or more in hot weather or during physical activity). When your water intake does not equal your output, you can become dehydrated.

This fluid does not have to be water alone. It can also be obtained from juice, milk, soup, and foods high in water such as fruits and vegetables. Caffeine-containing beverages (coffee, tea, cola) don't count because caffeine is a diuretic, making us lose water. A great plus for water in comparison to the other fluids is that it hydrates our body without extra calories and helps you feel full.

A Healthy Diet

A healthy diet is a diet that provides the nutrients your body needs in sufficient amounts. It helps us maintain or improve overall health. Different people need different amounts of calories and nutrients.

If you have a disease, your dietitian will guide you and make a proper meal plan that suits your health condition.

Here are guidelines for building a healthy diet that apply to all people and more importantly, to diabetics:

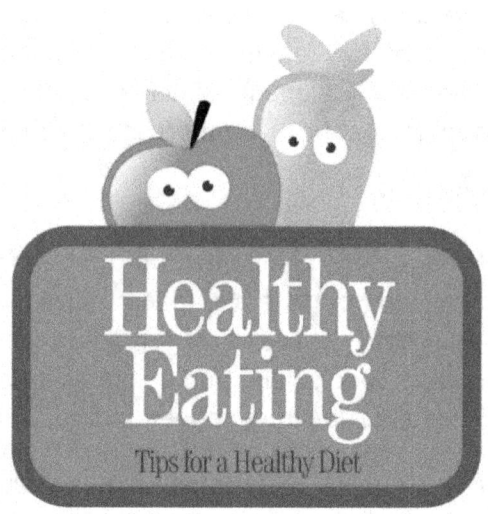

1. Start your day with a cup of warm water on an empty stomach.

2. Eat regularly three meals a day and 2 snacks and don't skip any meal.

3. Drink 2 to 3 liters of water daily.

4. Consume a Variety of Foods. No single category of food can give you all the nutrients you need. A healthy diet always includes food from each of the different food groups.

5. Eat the amount of food your body needs and keep an eye on portions. When you eat more food than your body needs, the extra calories are stored as fat. Find your ideal weight and activity level, and strive to reach and keep that weight.

6. Base each of your meals on a complex carbohydrate, such as oat, whole wheat, barley, wholemeal bread or brown rice, and include vegetables. Use high fiber wholegrain cereals as part of your breakfast, and use wholemeal bread for your toast. Whole grains retain the bran and germ and thus all (or nearly all) of the nutrients and fiber of the grain.

7. For lunch, choose lean protein, such as fish or chicken, with only a small amount of carbohydrate to get you through the afternoon.

8. Include green, orange, red, blue/purple and yellow produce like vegetables, fruits and legumes. The nutrients, fiber and other compounds in these foods may help protect against certain types of cancer and other diseases. Dietitians recommend plant foods because they include few calories and a lot of fiber, vitamins and minerals. In addition, they have no cholesterol and are low in fat.

9. Eat a diet low in fat and cholesterol. Less than 30% of the calories eaten by diabetics should come from fat.

10. Consume certain foods and drinks in moderation and limit highly processed foods. Carbohydrates, specifically candy, desserts, sweetened drinks, salt, and alcohol, should be consumed in moderation.

11. Cut down on the amount of refined white flour products in your diet, such as white bread, pizza and white pasta and rice. The refining process produces simple carbohydrates that aren't suitable for diabetics and many vitamins and minerals are lost.

12. Grill or boil instead of frying.

13. Eat fish and nuts and vegetable oils (canola and olive oil) and protect yourself from heart diseases because of its omega-3 polyunsaturated fats. Choose lean meats, skinless poultry and nonfat or low-fat dairy products.

14. Cut down on animal fat. Saturated fats, especially from red meat and processed meat, boost LDL (bad cholesterol).

15. Watch your calcium and vitamin D. Recommended calcium levels are 1000 mg per day, 1200 mg if you are over 50 years old. Try to get as much from food as possible from low-fat or nonfat dairy products and fortified foods such as soy products, broccoli, spinach, and almonds. It's hard to consume enough vitamin D from foods, and getting it from sunlight is risky. Many people—especially those who are over 60, live at northern latitudes or have darker skin—may need a D supplement (800 to 1,000 IU a day).

16. Keep sodium down, potassium up. People over 50 and those with hypertension, diabetes or chronic kidney disease should limit sodium to 1,500 milligrams a day because excess sodium raises blood pressure. At the same time, consume more potassium, which lowers blood pressure.

17. Refrain from smoking and drinking alcohol which increase the risk of diseases.

18. Prepare more of your own meals. Cooking more meals at home can help you take charge of what you're eating and better monitor exactly what goes into your food.

19. Read food labels.

20. Enjoy your food and chew it slowly.

My Plate

My Plate is a guide for healthy eating that suggests eating a variety of food while eating the appropriate amount from each group of food.

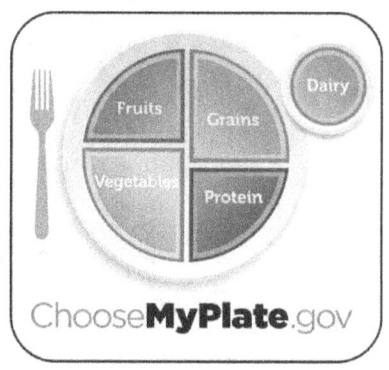

My Plate created by the US Department of Agriculture has 5 colors. Each color represents a food group. The larger the area of the color category, the more servings you need from this food group.

Grains (Orange), Vegetables (Green), Fruits (Red), Dairy (Blue), Proteins (Purple).

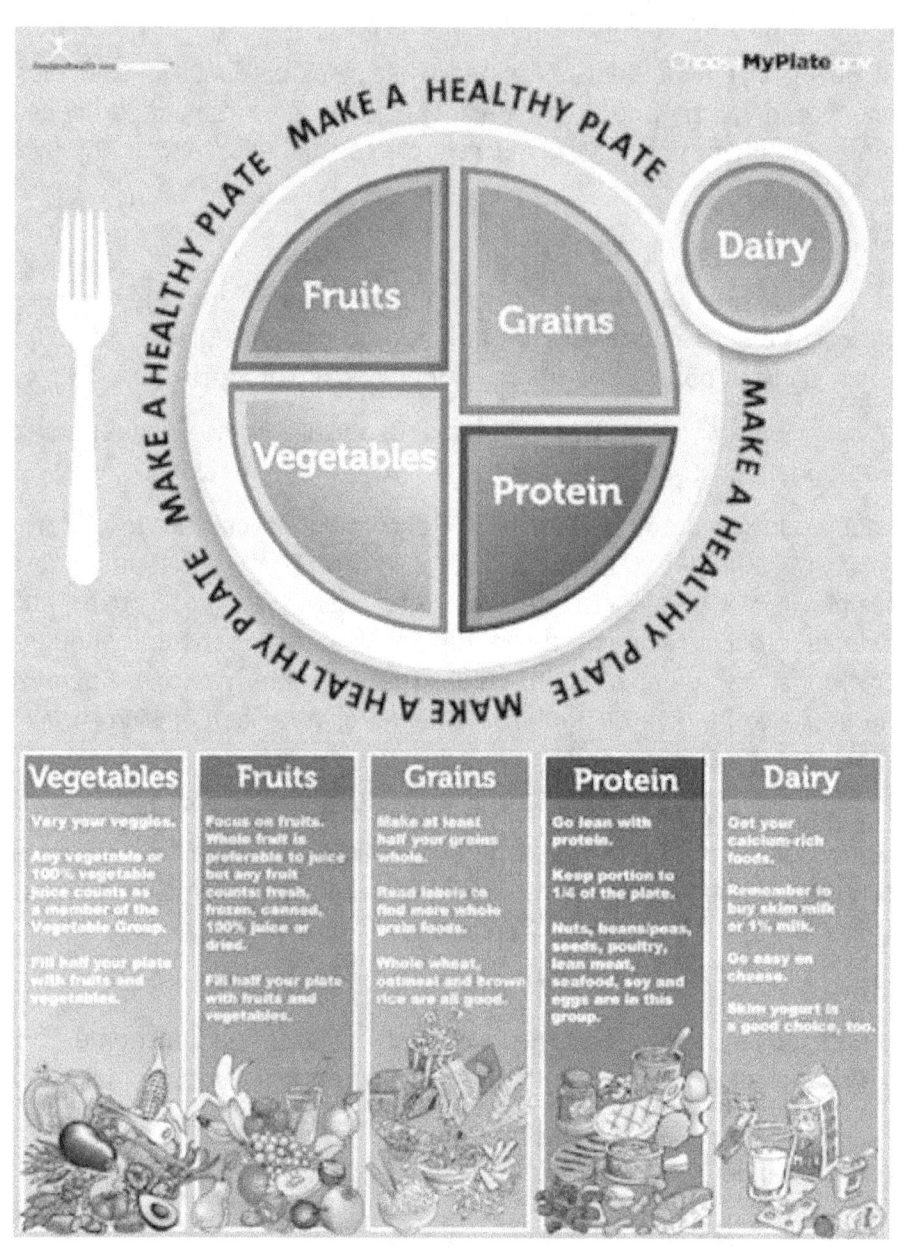

Here is an example of a healthy 2000 Kcal diabetes meal plan

Day 1	
Breakfast:	1 poached egg topped with parsley, 1 tsp olive oil and diced tomato on 1 slice sourdough toast + 1 cup of low fat milk.
Snack:	2 small pears.
Lunch:	Fish filet with tomato sauce: 90 gr grilled fish filet with 2 tbsp tomato sauce. Served with 150 gr brown rice with steamed broccoli and asparagus.
Snack:	Clean smoothie (1 cup kale, 1 cup coconut water (or just water), 1/2 cup apple, ¼ cup fresh mint leaves, juice of 1 lime), blend ingredients until smooth and add 1 tsp ground flax seeds.
Dinner:	Lentil-Avocado salad: Mixed Lettuce – 3 slices avocado – 30 gr lentil – fresh mushroom – tomatoes Lemon – 1 tsp olive oil.

Day 2	
Breakfast:	1 cup f plain yogurt + ½ cup oat + 6 strawberries + 1tsp flax seeds.
Snack:	1 cup of orange juice + 6 almonds.
Lunch:	90 g grilled chicken drizzled with lemon juice on a bed of 1 cup whole grain rice and steamed broccoli with artichoke.
Snack:	1 cup of soya milk.
Dinner:	2 cups veggie Soup (seasonal veggies - mushroom -onion - garlic – water - celery - 1 tsp canola oil- sea salt - pepper).

Day 3	
Breakfast:	Mozzarella, tomato & basil Omelet: 1 egg - 30 gr mozzarella cheese, tomato, basil, salt, pepper, 1 tsp sunflower oil. Served with cucumber and 1 slice whole grain toast.
Snack:	3 small carrots with lemon juice + 2 medium plums
Lunch:	90 g grilled lamb cutlets with steamed vegetables. 1 small grilled sweet potato.
Snack:	4 medium celery sticks + 1 cup of low fat milk
Dinner:	Salad of mixed lettuce, tomato , onion, lemon, 1 tsp olive oil, 1 tsp chia seeds. Mix all the chopped ingredients together

Day 4	
Breakfast:	2 cups low-fat goat milk blended with 16 small strawberries & + ½ cup oat.
Snack:	1 small apple.
Lunch:	Lentil soup – 50 gr dried red lentil mixed with 2 clove garlic,1 tbsp dried brown rice, 1 small chopped onion, 1 tsp dried thyme ,2 tsp cumin powder,1 tsp curry, salt and paper,1 tsp canola oil and 500 ml meat stock.
Snack:	1 cup of green tea with 1 small piece (40 gr) of dark chocolate
Dinner:	Tuna Mixed Beans salad with carrot: 90 gr tuna- 50 gr red beans- carrot- tomatoes-1 tsp olive oil- lemon juice-dill- broccoli, 1 tbsp lemon mustard.

Day 5	
Breakfast:	Turkey in brown baguette: 1 medium Baguette – 4 slices turkey – rocca – tomato-1 tsp sunflower seeds, 1 tsp mayo with mustard.
Snack:	1 cup of plain yogurt + 1 small apple.
Lunch:	Squash, eggplant, marrow and mushrooms. Cut the veggies into slices and add 1 tsp oil, salt and pepper and cook it in the oven. Served with 150 gr cup cooked quinoa.
Snack:	1 big peach + cucumber.
Dinner:	Salad of White & red cabbage, carrot, lemon, 1 tsp olive oil, 1 tsp hemp seeds. Mix all the chopped ingredients together and add 60 gr red beans.

Day 6	
Breakfast:	3 slices whole wheat bread with 60 g ricotta + 1 apple
Snack:	1 cup plain yogurt + 1 small apple
Lunch:	Chicken pesto sauce with vegetables ratatouille: 120 gr chicken breast without skin +2 tsp pesto sauce + 200 gr rice Ratatouille (cut the veggies into small pieces): carrot – marrow – mushroom - eggplant – salt – pepper + 2 tsp corn oil
Snack:	Clean smoothie (1 cucumber, 1 cup of kale, 1 cup of spinach, 1 cup of romaine lettuce , 4 celery stalks, 1 cup of coconut water), blend ingredients until smooth and add 1 tsp chia seeds. 10 pistachio.
Dinner:	Salad of Mixed lettuce, kale, cabbage, parsley, cucumbers, vinegar, lemon, 1 tsp olive oil, 1 tsp chia seeds.

Day 7	
Breakfast:	1 cup muesli with ½ cup blueberries, 1 tsp chia seeds, 1/2 cup oat, 1 cup low fat milk.
Snack:	1 medium grapefruit with 4 walnut halves.
Lunch:	2 cups mixed beans: 2 cups (white, red and black beans)- onions - whole garlic pieces - salt - sweet pepper - Canola oil – ginger powder- rosemary. 2 cups mixed beans: Heat 1 cup of water, add onion – 3 whole garlic pieces - salt - sweet pepper – 1 tsp canola oil – ginger powder- rosemary. Then add 2cups (white, red and black beans).
Snack:	30 gr low fat cheese + 2 carrots.
Dinner:	Salad of kale, mixed lettuce, parsley, cucumbers, lemon, carrot, fresh mushroom, 1 tsp olive oil, 1 tbsp sunflower seeds.

Glycemic Index and Diabetes

The glycemic index, or GI, measures how a carbohydrate-containing food raises blood glucose. Foods are ranked based on how they compare to a reference food — either glucose or white bread.

A food with a high GI raises blood glucose more than a food with a medium or low GI.

Meal planning with the GI involves choosing foods that have a low or medium GI. If eating a food with a high GI, you can combine it with low GI foods to help balance the meal, ADA recommends.

According to ADA, some examples of carbohydrate-containing foods with a low GI include dried beans and legumes (like kidney beans and lentils), all non-starchy vegetables, some starchy vegetables like sweet potatoes, most fruit, and many whole grain breads and cereals (like barley, whole wheat bread, rye bread, and all-bran cereal).

Meats and fats don't have a GI because they do not contain carbohydrate.

Below are examples of foods based on their GI.

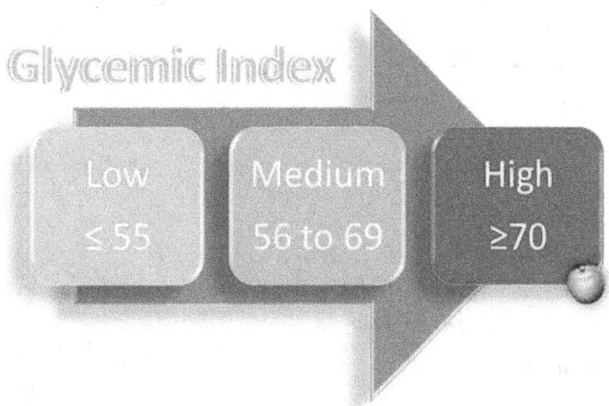

Low GI Foods (55 or less)

- 100% stone-ground whole wheat or pumpernickel bread
- Oatmeal (rolled or steel-cut), oat bran, muesli
- Pasta, converted rice, barley, bulgar
- Sweet potato, corn, yam, lima/butter beans, peas, legumes and lentils
- Most fruits, non-starchy vegetables and carrots

Medium GI (56-69)

- Whole wheat, rye and pita bread
- Quick oats
- Brown, wild or basmati rice, couscous

High GI (70 or more)

- White bread or bagel
- Corn flakes, puffed rice, bran flakes, instant oatmeal
- Shortgrain white rice, rice pasta, macaroni and cheese from mix
- Russet potato, pumpkin
- Pretzels, rice cakes, popcorn, saltine crackers
- melons and pineapple

Fruit Glycemic Index

Low GI 55 or less	Apples	Apricots	Banana
	Cherries	Grapefruit	Strawberries
	Kiwi fruit	Mango	Oranges
	Peach	Pears	Plums
	Persimmon		
Medium GI 56 - 69	Apricots, dried	Oranges	papaya
	Pineapple	Raisins	
High GI 70 or more	Banana (South Africa)	Dates, dried	melons
	Watermelon	Figs	Grapes

Be Active!

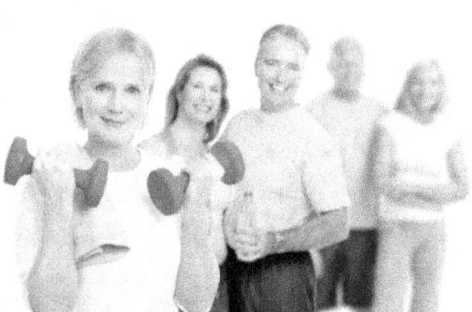

- Exercise burns extra body fat, which will help you lose weight or maintain a healthy weight. It also strengthens your muscles and bones.
- It cuts LDL and raises HDL.
- Regular exercise can help your body respond to insulin and is known to be effective in managing blood glucose.
- Exercise can improve your blood flow and circulation and raises your heart rate counts, especially in your arms and legs, where people with diabetes can have problems.
- For most people with diabetes, walking is a great choice. If you have foot problems from diabetes, your doctor may recommend minimizing the time you spend on your feet.
- Try new activities you have always wanted to try or something you enjoyed in the past like sports, dancing, yoga, walking, and swimming.

Exercising Safely

➢ Talk to your doctor first before starting an exercise routine and let him/her know what you want to do. Your doctor and dietitian will check to see if you need to change your meals, insulin, or diabetes medicines.

➢ Check your blood sugar before, during, or after exercise. If you plan to work out for more than an hour, check your blood sugar levels regularly during your workout, so you'll know if you need a snack. Check your blood sugar after every workout, so that you can adjust if needed.

➢ Hydrate. Drink water before, during, and after exercise.

➢ Ease into it. If you're not active now, start with 10 minutes of exercise at a time. Gradually work up to 30 minutes a day.

➢ Protect your feet. Check and clean it daily and wear athletic shoes that are the right type for your activity.

➢ Watch your body temperature.

➢ Exercise, eat, and take your medicines at the same time each day to prevent low blood sugar (hypoglycemia).

➢ Wear a medical identification tag.

➢ Always keep a handy snack like fruit or a fruit drink, on hand in case your blood sugar gets low.

➢ Check your ketones either by urine test or breath test and don't exercise if your ketones level is high.

➢ Carry a card that says you have diabetes, just in case.

Conclusion

Diabetes is the fastest growing long term disease that affects millions of people worldwide. In the United States 25.8 million people or 8.3% of the population have diabetes. Of these, 7.0 million have undiagnosed diabetes. In 2010, about 1.9 million new cases of diabetes were diagnosed in population over 20 years. It is said that if this trend continues, 1 in 3 Americans would be diabetic by 2050.

Healthy eating, being active, medicine, and tracking your blood sugar are the 4 cornerstones of diabetes care. Managing diabetes may feel like a huge task, but if you know how to control it and follow the previous information and educate yourself, it will be an easy and you will avoid too much pain. Another important part of diabetes management is reducing other cardiovascular disease risk factors, such as high blood pressure, obesity, high cholesterol and tobacco use.

Physical activity, diet, and appropriate use of insulin and oral medications help you lower blood sugar levels, alleviate symptoms, minimize or prevent long-term complications and save your life.

In recent years diabetes has been widely reported in the media and there is a heightened awareness of it than before, so people may be diagnosed earlier than before and the recent changes in the way diabetes is diagnosed have also made it easier to diagnose diabetes. Everyone has the risk factors should do diabetes test to protect himself especially from type 2 which we can control it and reverse it if he is in prediabetes stage.

Talk with your doctor and dietitian to get a better sense of your risk. They can help you make a plan that will keep you in good health.